Keto Diet Cookbook

Simple and Delicus Recipes with Easy Instruction and Ingredients

Caroline Smith

Trademarks that are mentioned are done without written consent and can in no way be considered an endorsement from the trademark holder.
DISCLAIMER

The content, writing, images, photos, descriptions and information contained in this book are for general guidance and are intended for informational purposes only for the readers.

The author has narrated his cooking and research experiences in this book by observing and evaluating relevant facts and figures. The author is not a registered dietitian and nutritional information in this book should only be used as a general guideline. Statements in this book have not been evaluated or approved by any regulatory authority.

The author has tried to provide all the information related to the ingredients, foods, and products, however, when certain ingredients get mixed, they may create some kind of cross-reaction which may cause allergy among some people. There may be products that will not be gluten-free and may contain ingredients that may cause a reaction. These products may include but are limited to, eggs, dairy, wheat, nuts, coconut, flour, soy, cocoa, milk, sugar, and other products. These may cause allergic reactions in some people due to cross-contamination from allergen-causing products.

The readers and purchasers of this book understand and consent that there may be ingredients in the foods which may contain certain allergens and the readers and purchasers hereby disclaimer the author of this book from all liabilities related to allergic and cross food reactions.

—

Table of Contents

Here Is Handy Tabular Conversion Chart

1 teaspoon = 1/3 tablespoon = 1/6 fluid ounce

1 tablespoon = 3 teaspoons = ½ fluid oz. = 1/16 cup

1 fluid ounce = 6 tsp. = 2 tbs = 1/8 cup = 1/16 pint

1 cup = 48 tsp. =16 tbs. =8 fluid oz. =½ pint = ¼ quart

1 pint = 16 fluid oz. = 2 cups = ½ quart.

1 quart = 32 fluid oz. = 4 cups = 2 pints

1 bottle is 750ml

Vegetable Omelette

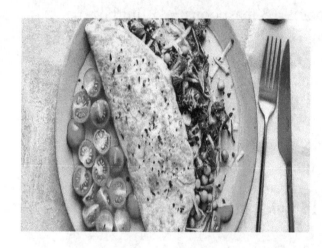

Prep Time: 5 minutes
Cook Time: 15 minutes
Serving: 1

Ingredients

- 1 cup of half sized cherry tomatoes
- 2 tablespoons of white vinegar
- 2 tablespoons of extra virgin olive oil
- 1 minced garlic clove
- 1 grated courgette
- Handful of kale
- 1 cup of frozen peas
- ⅛ teaspoon of red chilli flakes
- 2 golden eggs whisked

Directions

- Take a bowl add the half sized cherry tomatoes then add the white vinegar and sprinkle some seasonings. Toss all the ingredients together until well combined and then set them aside
- Take a nonstick pan, add the olive oil then add the minced garlic clove and let it saute for 2 minutes until its fragrance comes out. Then add the courgette and cook it for 5 minutes until it absorbs it's moisture
- Then add the kale and peas let it cook for about 4 minutes until kale is wilted
- Then season with some salt and red pepper flakes.
- Take a nonstick pan drizzle some olive oil then add the whisked eggs seasoned with the seasonings and cook it for 5 minutes then pile the cooked veggies in one side of the omellete and then fold on the one side
- Put the cooked omellete in a plate and serve with the cherry tomatoes
- Enjoy

Masala Omelette

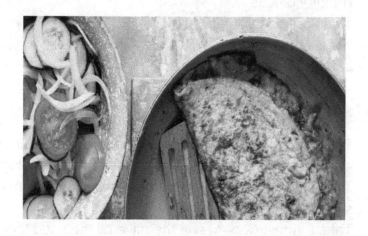

Prep Time: 10 minutes
Cook Time: 20 minutes
Serving: 2

Ingredients

- 1 tablespoon of extra virgin olive oil
- 1 small onion finely chopped
- 1 green chilli deseeded and sliced
- 1 long thumb sliced ginger finely chopped
- 1 teaspoon of whole spice powder
- ½ teaspoon of turmeric powder

Salad Ingredients

- 2 place sized ripe tomatoes cut into half sized
- Half cucumber thinly sliced
- 1 small sized onion thinly sliced
- 1 teaspoon of white wine vinegar

Directions

- First of all make a salad. Take a bowl add the salad ingredients and then add white wine vinegar and sprinkle some salt. Toss all the ingredients together until well combined
- Take a nonstick pan add the olive oil then add the sliced onions, chillies, ginger and tomatoes with a pinch of salt
- Let it cook for about 10 minutes until it is tender soft
- Then add the spices and let it cook for about 2 minutes more
- Take a bowl crack golden eggs beat them well and add the chopped coriander stir then to combine well
- Pour the egg in the pan and let it cook for about 5 minutes by flipping from both sides until it is totally cooked

- Then cut then into two halves and put it in a plate and serve with a salad
- Enjoy

Chargrilled Steak With Chopped Salad

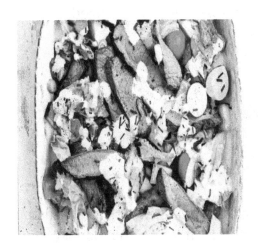

Prep Time: 10 minutes
Cook Time: 20 minutes
Servings: 2 people

Ingredients

- 1 teaspoon of extra virgin olive oil
- 3 rump steaks
- ½ teaspoon of smoked paprika
- 1 teaspoon of garlic salt
- ¼ teaspoon of freshly ground black pepper
- 2 chopped spring onions
- 6 radishes, cut into half sized
- 2 little gems cut into bite-sized chunks
- 10-12 cherry tomatoes cut into half sized
- ½ cucumber thinly sliced

Blue Cheese Dressing

- 5 tablespoons of sour cream
- 50 grams of creamy blue cheese

Directions

- Take a plate put the steak then rub the oil on both sides. Then spread them garlic salt, paprika, and pepper. Then rub them on both sides
- Now make a cheese dressing. Take a bowl put the sour cream, and then add the cheese. Mash them together
- Then add the vinger, mustard and water stir them to combine all the ingredients together until well combined
- Take a nonstick pan and sprinkle some oil then put the steak on the pan and cook them for 5 minutes by flipping from both sides
- Take a bowl add the salad vegetables toss them to combine
- Then plate them with a steak. Then drizzle the dressing and sprinkle the chives

- Then serve them and enjoy

Crunchy Veggies and Smoked Tofu Salad

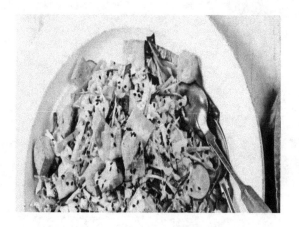

Prep Time: 10 minutes
Cook Time: 25 minutes
Servings: 2 people

Ingredients

- 2 small sized carrots peeled and shredded
- 150 grams of Chinese cabbage shredded
- 5 radishes peeled a d sliced
- 4 spring onions, peeled and shredded
- 1 teaspoon of rice vinegar
- 200 grams of smoked tofu block cut into cube

Sesame Dressing Ingredients

- 2 tablespoons of tahini sauce
- 1 tablespoon of Mirin
- 1 tablespoon of soy sauce

Directions

- Take a bowl add the shredded carrots, shredded cabbage, onions, sliced cucumbers and sliced radishes. Pour the white wine vinegar and sprinkle some salt. Toss all the ingredients together until well combined and then leave them for 10 minutes
- Now take a bowl add the sesame dressing ingredients and whisk them by adding water to make them thin dressing
- Now take a nonstick pan add the olive oil then put the sliced tofu
- Let them dry until it turns golden brown and crispy
- Then add the spinach to the veggies toss everything together with the dressing
- Top them with the tofu, sesame seeds and the rest of the dressings
- Then serve them and enjoy

Omelette Irani

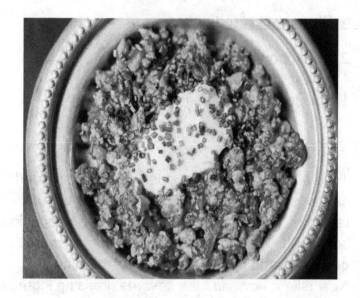

Prep Time: 10 minutes
Cook Time: 15 minutes
Serving: 2

Ingredients

- 2 tablespoons of extra virgin olive oil
- 1 minced garlic clove
- 1 small sized onion finely chopped
- 6 plum tomatoes deseeded and chopped
- 2 tablespoons of tomato puree
- 6 golden eggs
- 2 tablespoons of unsalted melted butter
- 2 tablespoons of chives finely chopped

Directions

- Take a nonstick pan add the extra virgin olive oil and then add the minced garlic clove. Let it cook for about 2 minutes until its fragrance comes out
- Then add the onions and let them cook until they are tendered
- After that add the tomato puree and stir them to combine
- Let them cook for about 5 minutes then turn off the flame
- Take a bowl crack the golden eggs and whisk them together until well combined
- Then slowly pour the egg mixture in the tomato puree pan and turn on the flame stir them continuously until they are well combined together
- Stir the eggs until they are totally set
- Then transfer this cooked eggs in a serving plate then drizzle some unsalted melted butter and sprinkle some chives
- Then serve them with any of your favorite bread and enjoy

Keto Breakfast Recipes

Soft Boiled Duck Eggs With Bacon And Asparagus Soldiers

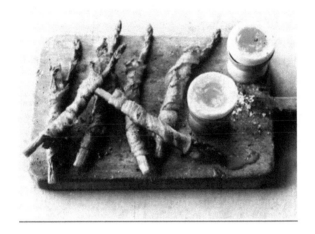

Preparing Time: 5 minutes,
Cooking Time: 25 minutes
Serving: 2 people's

Ingredients

- 8 asparagus with ends removed
- 4 long slices of thin rustic bread (preferably sourdough)
- 8 strips of bacon
- 4 duck eggs

Directions

- Heat up the grill, remove the ends of the asparagus. Cut the bread into 12 soldiers, shorter than the asparagus
- Place the spear onto each soldier wrap tightly with a rasher of bacon
- Grill them for 15 minutes until the bacon is crisp
- Pour the 3 cups of water in the pan and dip the eggs in the water and let them boil for 8 minutes.
- After 8 minutes cut the eggs into 2 half and then serve them immediately with the warm soldiers for dipping

Keto Green Eggs

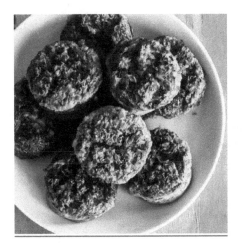

Preparing Time: 15 minutes,
Cooking Time: 40 minutes
Serving: 4 people's

Ingredients

- 1 cup of finely chopped broccoli
- 10 eggs beaten / whisked
- 10-12 slices of ham, diced
- 1 onion finely chopped
- ½ cup of coconut milk
- Some kosher salt to taste
- Some ground black pepper to taste
- 1 teaspoon of baking powder

Directions

- Preheat the oven at 180 F
- Take a bowl add all the ingredients together mix them together until well combined
- Take silicone muffin trays spray with some olive oil
- Pour the batter in the silicone muffin cups
- Bake it for 30 minutes
- Serve them at room temperature and Enjoy

Sprout & Spinach Baked Eggs

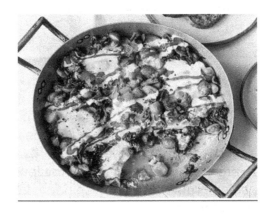

Preparing Time: 10 minutes,
Cooking Time: 20 minutes
Serving: 2 people's

Ingredients

- 2 tablespoons of extra-virgin olive oil
- 1 tablespoon of cumin seeds
- 1 finely chopped onion
- 2 minced garlic cloves
- 1 green chilli
- 300 grams of Brussels sprouts roughly shredded
- 500 grams of baby spinach
- 2 tablespoon of lemon juice
- 6 golden eggs
- Sriracha dip for serving

Directions

- Heat the oil in a frying pan, then add cumin seeds, stir them for 1 minute. Then add chopped onions, garlic cloves, green chilli, stir all the ingredients continuously until they are well combined for 5 minutes. Then add the Brussels sprouts and baby spinach. Let them wilted down for 4 minutes
- Pour the lemon juice and stir them continuously until they are tendered or well combined
- When Brussels sprouts and baby spinach is cooked make 6 holes in the pan and crack 6 golden eggs and cook them for 7 minutes
- Then sprinkle some chopped coriander. Then drizzled with some yogurt
- Enjoy6

Keto Breakfast Burritos

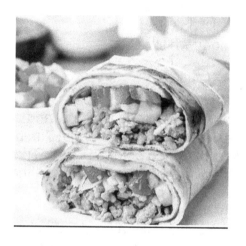

Preparing Time: 10 minutes,
Cooking Time: 25 minutes
Serving: 2 people's

Ingredients

- 1 pound of chopped sausages
- 1 cup of chopped cucumbers
- 1 cup of peeled and diced tomatoes
- 1 onion chopped
- Some kosher salt to taste
- Some ground black pepper to taste
- 2 teaspoons of extra virgin olive oil
- Some chopped parsley
- Pinch of chilli powder
- 8 golden eggs whisked

Directions

- Take a nonstick pan, add olive oil, and add chopped sausages, let them cook for about 7 minutes until they are cooked or turned golden brown. Then add some salt and black pepper to taste. Stir all the ingredients together until well combined
- Turn off the flame.
- Prepare the salsa, take a bowl, add chopped cucumbers, diced tomatoes, and chopped onions. Then add some salt and black pepper to taste
- Stir all the ingredients together until well combined
- Take a bowl crack 8 golden eggs , chopped parsley whisked them together until well combined
- Take another pan add 1 teaspoon of olive oil pour the whisked egg slowly and form 8 egg wraps
- Put the egg wraps on the wooden tray and add some sausages, then add the salsa slightly wrap the egg rolls and serve them with your favorite sauce and enjoy

Raspberry, Almond & Oat Breakfast Cookies

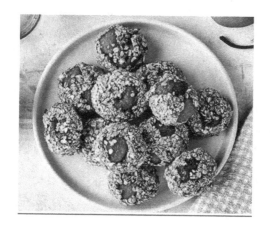

Preparing Time: 10 minutes,
Cooking Time: 20 minutes
Serving: 4 people's

Ingredients

- 3 ripe bananas
- 150 grams of oats
- 3 tablespoons of ground almonds
- ½ teaspoon of cinnamon powder
- 100 grams of raspberries

Directions

- Preheat the air fryer basket lined with parchment paper at 400 degrees
- Take a bowl, add ripe bananas, oats, ground almonds, cinnamon powder and raspberries. Mix all the ingredients carefully so that the raspberries should not break
- Now take a wooden spoon and take a thick batter, make the balls of this batter by using your hands
- Put these balls on the parchment paper and cook them for about 15 minutes until they are turned into crispy and golden brown
- Remove from the air fryer basket and let them cool
- Serve them and enjoy

Tropical Breakfast Bars

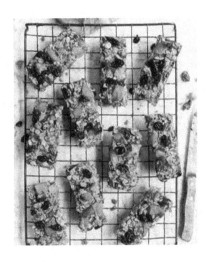

Preparing Time: 15 minutes,
Cooking Time: 40 minutes
Serving: 5 people's

Ingredients

- 2 tablespoons of extra virgin olive oil and some extra for the tin
- 3 large ripe bananas
- 1 golden egg whisked
- 1 cup of brown sugar
- 250 grams of nutty muesli
- 1 cup of mixed dry fruits

Directions

- Take a bowl, add ripe bananas, then add olive oil, beaten egg and sugar.
- Mix all the ingredients together until well combined. Then add nutty muesli and tropical dry fruits mix then by using your hands
- Now spoon this mixture in the tin sprayed with some olive oil then sprinkle some tropical dry fruits
- Let them cook for about 35 minutes and after cooking let them cool and slice them in bars
- Serve them and enjoy

Two-minutes Keto Breakfast Smoothie

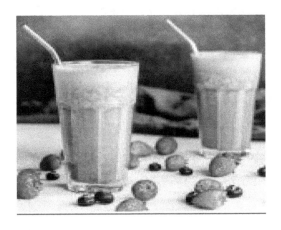

Preparing Time: 2 minutes,
Cooking Time: 5 minutes
Serving: 2 people's

Ingredients

- 1 cup of frozen berries
- 1 cup frozen avocados
- 5 leaves of baby spinach
- ¼ teaspoon of cocoa powder
- 1 tablespoon of nut butter
- 3 tablespoons of nut milk
- 1 glass of water
- ½ teaspoon of collagen powder
- ½ teaspoon of protein powder
- ⅛ teaspoon of chia seeds
- 1 teaspoon of coconut powder

Directions

- Take a blender and add all ingredients in the blender and blend it until a smooth creamy smoothie formed

Keto Breakfast Sandwiches

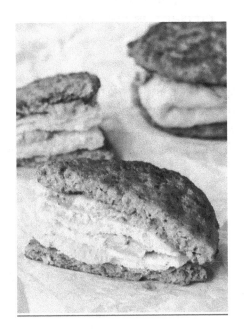

Preparing Time: 15 minutes,
Cooking Time: 15 minutes
Serving: 2 people's

Ingredients

- 2 sausage patties
- 1 golden egg
- 1 tablespoon of cream cheese
- 3 tablespoons of cheddar cheese
- ½ avocado sliced
- 1 tablespoon of sriracha dip
- Some kosher salt to taste
- Some ground black pepper to taste

Directions

- Take a nonstick pan, cook the sausage patties on medium heat until cooked
- Take a bowl and add cream cheese and cheddar cheese. Microwave them for about 1 minutes then remove it from the oven
- Add stomachs dip in the cheese mixture and then set aside
- Take a bowl crack eggs and add seasonings and whisk them
- Pour this egg on the pan and make an omelette
- Remove the omelette in the pan spread sriracha dip and cheese mixture assemble them with the sausage patties
- Enjoy

keto Friendly Double Chocolate Smoothie

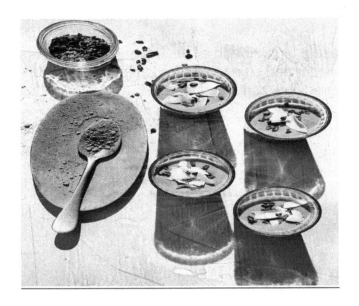

Preparing Time: 3 minutes,
Cooking Time: 2 minutes
Serving: 2 people's

Ingredients

- 1 ripe avocado peeled and diced
- 1 tablespoon of cocoa powder
- 3 tablespoons of keto-friendly chocolate protein powder
- ½ teaspoon of chia seeds
- ¼ cup of coconut milk
- 4 cups of almond milk

Directions

- Take a blender add all the ingredients together in a blender and blend them for 2 minutes until all the ingredients combined together

Keto Blueberry Muffins

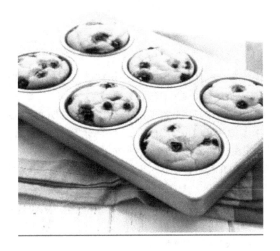

Preparing Time: 15 minutes,
Cooking Time: 35 minutes
Serving: 4 people's

Ingredients

- 1 container (5 ounces) of Greek yogurt
- 3 large golden eggs
- ½ teaspoon of vanilla extract
- Some salt to taste
- 3 cups of almond flour
- ⅓ cup of any sweetener of your choice
- 2 tablespoons of baking powder
- Some water to thin if needed
- ½ cup of fresh blueberries

Directions

- Preheat the air fryer basket lined with the silicone muffin tray at 325 degrees
- Take a blender add vanilla extract, eggs, yogurt and some salt in the blender. Blender them until all the ingredients are blend together very well
- Then add flour, sweetener and baking powder and blend them again until well combined
- Then add some water in the blender and mix the batter by using spoon
- Stir the batter in the silicone muffin cups and bake them for about 30 minutes. And then remove from the silicone tray and serve them
- Enjoy

Keto Pancakes

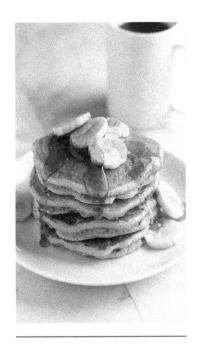

Preparing Time: 10 minutes,
Cooking Time: 15 minutes
Serving: 4 people's

Ingredients

- 1 cup of almond flour
- ½ cup of coconut flour
- 3 tablespoons of any sweetener of your choice
- 1 teaspoon of baking powder
- ½ cup of almond milk
- ¼ cup of coconut oil
- Some sea salt to taste
- 1 teaspoon of vanilla extract
- Some honey to drizzle on-the-go pancakes
- Some butter cut into cubes

Directions

- Take a bowl add all the ingredients together until thick batter is formed to make pancakes
- Take a nonstick pan, drizzle some coconut oil, pour the batter and circle them and make the pancakes. Cook them until bubbles starts to form and pancakes turned into golden brown
- Remove the pancakes in the plate put cubed butter, then drizzle some honey on the top
- Serve them and enjoy

Keto Hot Chocolate

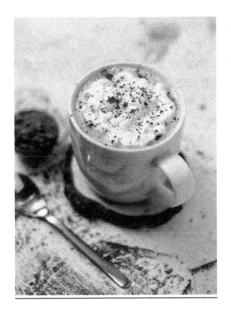

Preparing Time: 2 minutes,
Cooking Time: 6 minutes
Serving: 1 people

Ingredients

- 1 cup of unsweetened almond milk
- 3 tablespoons of heavy whipping cream
- 2 tablespoons of any sweetener of your choice
- 1 tablespoon of unsweetened cocoa powder

Directions

- Take a pan on medium heat
- Add all the ingredients and let them cook for 5 minutes
- Pour them in the cup top with heavy cream and sprinkle some cocoa powder and serve
- Enjoy

Keto Breakfast Cups

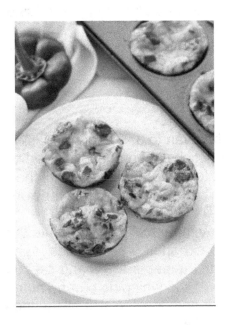

Preparing Time: 10 minutes,
Cooking Time: 25 minutes
Serving: 2 people's

Ingredients

- 10 golden eggs
- 8 slices of bacon
- 1 cup of finely chopped onion
- 1 green chilli finely chopped
- 1 cup of spinach finely chopped
- ½ cup of whipping cream
- 1 cup of grated cheddar cheese
- ½ cup of Monterey Jack cheese
- 1 tablespoon of Worcestershire sauce
- Some sea salt and black pepper to taste
- Some dash of nutmeg
- Some finely chopped fresh parsley
- Some red pepper flakes

Directions

- Preheat the oven to 375 degrees
- Take a nonstick pan, add thinly sliced bacon and let them cook for about 5 minutes until they are tender or turned into golden brown. Once they are fully cooked remove them in a plate
- In the remaining bacon grease saute the chopped onions and chopped green chillies for about 3 minutes
- Put them on the paper towel and set them aside
- Take a bowl, add whipping cream, nutmeg, sauce, pepper, salt and eggs. Whisk all the ingredients together until well combined
- Now take another bowl add pepper mixture and bacon mixture and then in the same bowl mix them
- Take a silicone muffin cups tray
- Add the Monterey Jack cheese and eggs mixture in each muffin cups
- Drizzle some crumbled bacon on each cup. Then sprinkle some finely chopped parsley and red pepper

- Bake them for about 20 minutes until they are tendered or cooked
- Serve them in a plate with any of your favorite sauce

Cabbage Hash Browns

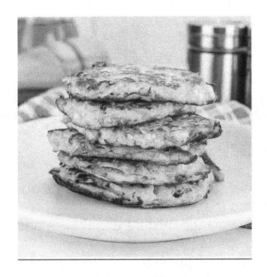

Preparing Time: 10 minutes,
Cooking Time: 15 minutes
Serving: 2 people's

Ingredients

- 3 golden eggs
- Some sea salt to taste
- Some ground white pepper to taste
- 2 tablespoons of extra virgin olive oil
- 7 ounces of cabbage
- 1 teaspoon of onion powder
- ½ teaspoon of ginger and garlic powder

Directions

- Finely shredded the cabbage using food processor
- Take a bowl add shredded cabbage, crack eggs, salt, pepper, onion powder, ginger and garlic powder in the bowl
- Mix all the ingredients together with the help of wooden spoon
- Take a nonstick pan turn on the flame and drizzle some olive oil on the pan
- Pour the cabbage mixture into 6 piles and press them by using spatula
- Cook them by flipping from both sides for 3 minutes, until they are tendered or golden brown
- Serve them with your favorite sauce and enjoy

Keto Cereal

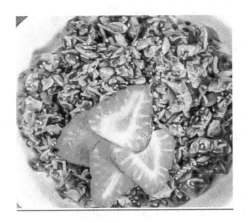

Preparing Time: 10 minutes,
Cooking Time: 40 minutes
Serving: 2 people's

Ingredients

- 1 cup of unsweetened coconut in shredded form
- 1 cup of unshaved coconut
- 1 cup of almond flakes
- 3 tablespoons of flaxseeds
- 3 tablespoons of pepitas
- 3 tablespoons of chia seeds
- 1 tablespoon of ground cinnamon powder
- 3 tablespoon of coconut oil
- ½ teaspoon of vanilla essence
- 2 tablespoons of Erythritol

Directions

- Preheat the air fryer basket lined with parchment paper at 325 degrees
- Take a bowl add all the ingredients together until well combined
- Spread these ingredients on the parchment paper and bake them for about 35 minutes
- Serve them after every 5 minutes to prevent them from burning
- Remove from the air fryer basket until they are turned into crispy and golden brown
- Allow them to add in the container and let them cool or serve it

Keto Lunch Recipes

Creamy Avocado Keto Chicken Salad

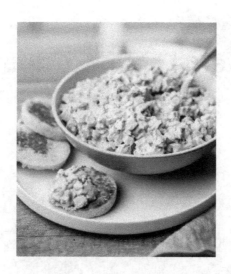

Preparing Time: 10 minutes,
Cooking Time: 10 minutes

Serving: 3 people's

Ingredients

- 3 cups of cooked chicken finely diced
- ⅓ cup of mayonnaise
- 1 medium-sized avocado peeled and chopped
- 1 stalk of celery finely chopped
- 1 small onion finely chopped
- 2 tablespoons of cilantro finely chopped
- 1 tablespoon of fresh Lemon juice
- Some kosher salt to taste
- Some ground black pepper to taste

Directions

- Take a food processor, add half of the avocado, mayonnaise, lemon juice, salt and black pepper. Process them into creamy form
- Now take a bowl add the rest of the half avocado peeled and diced, diced chicken, celery stalks and chopped onions. Stir them to combine all the ingredients together
- Now add the mayonnaise mixture on the top of the bowl full of the rest of the ingredients
- Now combine all the ingredients together until well combined
- Serve with your favorite keto bread and enjoy

Keto Popcorn Salad

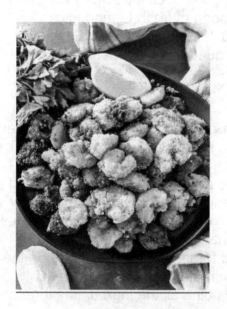

Preparing Time: 5 minutes,
Cooking Time: 10 minutes
Serving: 6 people's

Ingredients

- 1 lbs of shrimps
- 2 golden eggs
- ½ cup of coconut flour
- 1 tablespoon of Cajun spice blend
- Some kosher salt to taste
- ½ cup of the coconut oil for frying

Directions

- Take a nonstick skillet for frying add coconut oil in it
- Take a bowl crack golden eggs whisk them together until well combined
- Take another bowl add coconut flour, some kosher salt to taste and Cajun spice blend. Mix all the ingredients together until well combined
- Now dip the shrimp in the egg, then dip in the flour mixture. Then put in the nonstick skillet and let them fry

Keto Deviled Egg

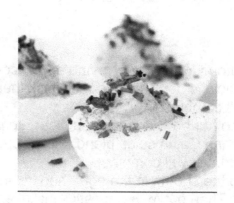

Preparing Time: 10 minutes,
Cooking Time: 8 minutes
Serving: 12 people's

Ingredients

- 6 golden eggs
- ¼ cup of mayonnaise
- 1 tablespoon of Dijon mustard sauce
- 1 tablespoon of apple cider vinegar
- ¼ teaspoon of garlic powder
- Some kosher salt to taste
- 5 slices of cooked bacon
- Some smoked paprika
- Freshly chopped chives for sprinkling

Directions

- Take a nonstick skillet and add water to it. Then add 6 golden eggs. Let them boil for about 10 minutes
- After 10 minutes peel them and place them in the bowl and let them cool
- Now slice the eggs in half of them. Then put out the egg yolk and mash them.
- Add mayonnaise, Dijon mustard, apple cider vinegar and garlic powder. Mix them by using a fork.
- Now pip the egg yolk back into the egg white. Sprinkle with some smoked paprika, crumbled bacon & fresh chives

Keto Macaroni Salad

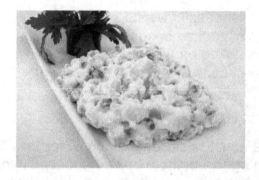

Preparing Time: 3 minutes,
Cooking Time: 10 minutes
Serving: 2 people's

Ingredients

- 1 cup of cauliflower florets cut into small pieces
- 2 tablespoons of sugar-free mayonnaise
- ½ tablespoon of apple cider vinegar
- Some kosher salt to taste
- Some ground black pepper to taste
- ⅓ teaspoon of stevia
- 1 tablespoon of Dijon mustard
- 2 tablespoons of celery stalks thinly chopped
- 2 tablespoons of chopped onions
- 2 tablespoons of grated carrots
- 2 tablespoons of chopped olives

Directions

- Take a double broiler and steam the cauliflower until tendered. Take a bowl add mayonnaise, salt, apple cider vinegar, Dijon mustard and sweetener.
- Mix them until well combined
- Take a large bowl add cauliflower, grated carrots, chopped onions, chopped olives, pepper and celery stalks. Stir them to combine well all the ingredients. Then pour the mayonnaise mixture on the salad and mix them
- Put them in the refrigerator for overnight and serve chilled
- Enjoy

Keto Tuna Salad

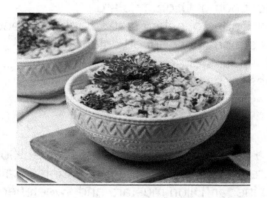

Preparing Time: 5 minutes,
Cooking Time: 10 minutes
Serving: 4 people's

Ingredients

- 10 ounces of tuna water drained
- 1 large avocado
- 1 rib of celery
- 2 cloves of garlic
- Some kosher salt to taste
- Some ground black pepper to taste
- ½ cucumber peeled and chopped
- ½ cup of parsley finely chopped
- 1 tablespoon of lemon juice
- 3 tablespoon of mayonnaise
- 1 small red onion finely chopped

Directions

- Drain the vegetables with water and let them dry with paper towel
- Then take a bowl add the vegetables and finely chopped them
- Now finely chopped the parsley and set then aside
- Take a bowl add the chopped veggies and then add the mashed avocado mix them well then sprinkle some ground black pepper and salt. Stir them to combine well
- Garnish then with the remaining chopped parsley and enjoy

Keto Egg Salad

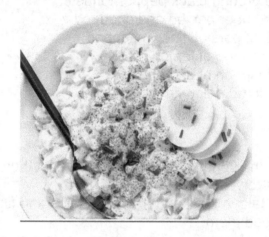

Preparing Time: 5 minutes,
Cooking Time: 0 minutes
Serving: 4 people's

Ingredients

- ½ cup of mayonnaise
- Some kosher salt to taste
- Some ground black pepper to taste
- 1 tablespoon of Dijon mustard
- 1 tablespoon of lemon juice
- 8 golden eggs diced
- 1 small onion finely chopped
- 1 stalk of celery finely chopped
- 2 tablespoons of chives finely chopped
- Finely chopped paprika finely chopped

Directions

- Take a bowl, add mayonnaise, lemon juice, and Dijon mustard. Stir them to combine well until smooth
- Take another bowl, add eggs and then add celery, onions and chives. Sprinkle some salt and black pepper. Pour the mayonnaise mixture and stir them to combine well and then sprinkle with some finely chopped paprika
- Serve them and enjoy

Keto Cobb Salad

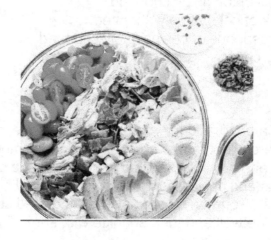

Preparing Time: 5 minutes,
Cooking Time: 0 minutes
Serving: 4 people's

Ingredients

- 4 cups of finely chopped lettuce
- 3 cups of watercress finely chopped
- 8 slices of cooked bacon (Crumbled)
- 2 large sized chicken breasts cut into cubes and shredded
- 2 cups of grape tomatoes cut into half sized
- Some kosher salt to taste
- Some ground black pepper to taste
- ½ cup of ranch dressing
- 2 tablespoons of chives finely chopped
- 2 avocados sliced
- 4 golden eggs boiled and sliced

Directions

- Take a bowl add all the ingredients except the dressing. Sprinkle some salt and black pepper
- Pour the dressing on the ingredients. Toss them to combine. Serve them and enjoy

Keto Broccoli Salad

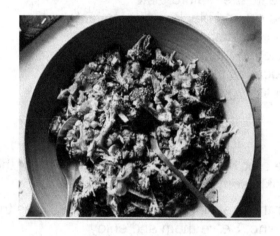

Preparing Time: 15 minutes,
Resting Time: 20 minutes
Serving: 4 people's

Ingredients

- 5 slices of bacon cooked and crumbled
- 3 cups of broccoli florets cut into 4 pieces
- ½ red onion diced
- ½ cup of chopped walnuts
- 1 cup of shredded cheddar cheese
- ¼ cup of sunflower seeds
- ¼ cup of sour cream
- 3 tablespoons of mayonnaise
- 2 teaspoons of apple cider vinegar
- 1 packet of any sweetener of your choice

Directions

- Take a nonstick pan add bacon, cook them until it turns crispy and crumbled
- Then remove them in a bowl and reserve the bacon fat for later use
- Take a bowl add mayonnaise, sour cream, apple cider vinegar, sweetener, and bacon fat. Stir them to combine well
- Take another bowl add broccoli, onion, walnuts, cheese, bacon and sunflower seeds
- Pour the dressing and toss them to combine well. Now allow the salad to rest for about 10 minutes
- Then serve them and enjoy

Keto Green Salad

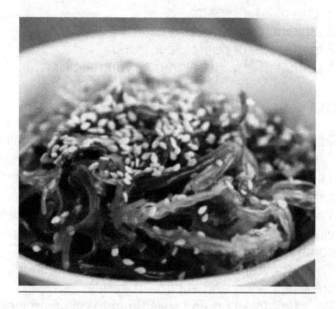

Preparing Time: 15 minutes,
Resting Time: 10 minutes
Serving: 4 people's

Ingredients
- 2 cups of lettuce hearts
- 1 bunch of asparagus
- 1 tablespoon of grape seed oil
- 2 tablespoons of pumpkin seeds
- Some kosher salt to taste

Ingredients For Garlic Dressing

- ½ cup of cashew
- 1 cup of water
- 1 tablespoon of lemon juice
- Some Himalayan salt to taste
- 1 teaspoon of garlic powder
- 1 tablespoon of nutritional yeast
- 1 tablespoon of mustard sauce

Directions

- Water drain the lettuce and then set aside
- Take a nonstick pan add pumpkin seeds and then roast them (Do it carefully and not burn them) then set aside then
- Now cut the asparagus into small pieces and carefully steam them by sprinkling some salt
- Then drain the asparagus with cold water. Then brush them with oil and grilled then in the grilling pan for 5 minutes carefully that they shouldn't be burned
- Now arrange the lettuce in the pan then arrange the slived avocados on the top of the lettuce leaves
- Then sprinkle the roasted pumpkin seeds and top them with asparagus
- Then drizzle some creamy garlic dressing
- Then sprinkle on then some grinned peppercorns
- Serve them and enjoy

Prawns & Buttermilk Dressing & Celery Salad

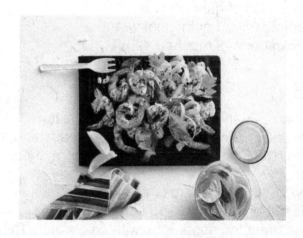

Preparing Time: 15 minutes,
Resting Time: 10 minutes
Serving: 4 people's

Ingredients

- 2 tablespoons of extra virgin olive oil
- 3 cloves of garlic minced
- 25 green prawns (Peeled and tails removed)
- 1 tablespoon of lemon juice
- 3 tablespoons of buttermilk
- 1 tablespoon of Dijon mustard
- 1 tablespoon of white vinegar
- 2 celery stalks or 1 cup of celery leaves
- 1 tablespoon of finely chopped chives
- 1 fennel bulb
- 1 cup of mint leaves

Directions

- First of all preheat barbecue grill. Take a bowl add prawns, lemon juice, olive oil and garlic. Stir them to combine well all the ingredients. Then dip the prawns in them. Let them marinate for about 1 hour until all the ingredients together well combined
- Take another bowl add Dijon mustard, vinegar, butter milk, olive oil and chives. Combine all the ingredients together until well combined
- Now cut the celery stalks into long strips
- Now thinly slice the fennel and toss them in the lemon juice. Then add celery stalks and mint leaves. Combine all the ingredients together until well combined
- Cook the prawns on the grill and then serve them with buttermilk dressings, celery salad and lemon wedges
- Serve them and Enjoy

Keto Grilled Chicken

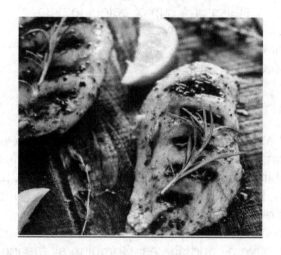

Preparing Time: 7 minutes,
Resting Time: 14 minutes
Serving: 4 people's

Ingredients

- 4 tablespoons of mayonnaise
- 2 tablespoons of coconut aminos
- 2 tablespoons of lemon juice
- 1 teaspoon of Lemon zest
- Some kosher salt to taste
- Some ground black pepper to taste
- ½ teaspoon of cayenne pepper
- 15 ounces of chicken breasts or thighs
- 1 teaspoon of rosemary powder
- 1 teaspoon of garlic powder
- 1 teaspoon of Dijon mustard

Directions

- Take a bowl add mayonnaise, lemon juice, lemon zest, Dijon mustard, salt, black pepper, cayenne pepper, garlic powder, rosemary powder, coconut aminos. Mix all the ingredients together until well combined
- Now divide the marinade into two bowls then spread half of the mayonnaise on 1 side of the chicken breast, and grill the chicken breast for 7 minutes then flip the side up then apply the rest of the mayonnaise on the flip side and let them cook for another 7 minutes at 155 degrees
- Then remove from the grill and serve them and enjoy

Keto Crispy Pork Belly Salad With Mint & Coriander

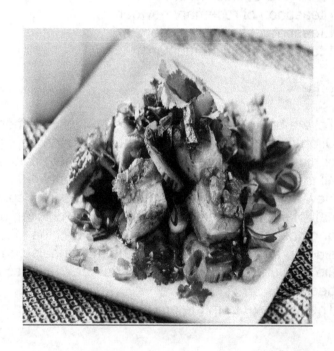

Preparing Time: 30 minutes,
Cooking Time: 1 minutes
Serving: 4 people's

Ingredients

- 1 kg of boneless belly pork
- 2 teaspoons Caster sugar
- 2 teaspoons Lemon juice
- 3 teaspoons Fish sauce
- 3 spring onions, finely sliced
- 1 small cucumber peeled thinly sliced
- 1 red chilli finely chopped with seeds removed
- ¼ cup of Mint leaves
- ¼ cup of Coriander leaves
- ¼ cup of Thai basil leaves
- ¼ cup of Salted and chopped peanuts

Directions

- Preheat the oven at 180 F
- Take a boneless belly pork. Dry them with the paper towel and let them dry.
- Now sprinkle some salt and microwave the belly pork for 2 hours by drizzling some water. When the pork is cooked remove them in a plate and let them dry
- Take a bowl, add fish sauce, sugar, lime juice, whisk them together until well combined. Then add the pork in the bowl. Then take a bowl and add spring onions, cucumber, chilli herbs, and toss them together.
- Then divide the salad among plates then scatter peanuts and serve
- Enjoy

Keto Bone Steaks With Mushrooms

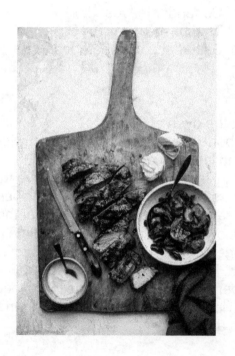

Preparing Time: 5 minutes,
Cooking Time: 20 minutes
Serving: 4 people's

Ingredients

- 1 lbs of steak (about 1 ½ inches thick)
- 4 teaspoons of unsalted melted butter
- 1 tablespoon of fresh minced garlic
- Some kosher salt to taste
- Some ground black pepper to taste

For The Mushrooms

- 2 cups of white mushrooms thinly sliced
- 2 tablespoons of unsalted melted butter
- 1 tablespoon of freshly minced garlic
- Some sea salt to taste

Directions

- Preheat the grill on high flame
- Till then dry them steak with a paper towel and then take a small bowl add unsalted melted butter, freshly minced garlic, some kosher salt to taste and black pepper to taste. Mix them until well combined
- Then brush them on one side of the steak and then on preheated grill put the butter side down on the grill
- Then spread the unsalted melted butter on the top side of the steak
- Cook the steak until it reaches the desired doneness. Place then in the plate and let them set aside till then prepare the mushrooms
- Take a bowl, add sliced mushrooms, unsalted butter, freshly minced garlic, some salt to taste and mix them well until well combined.
- Take 2 foils then place these mushrooms in these coils

then place them in the grill. Then grill them for 5 minutes
- Serve the mushrooms over the steak and enjoy

Keto Vegetable Frittata

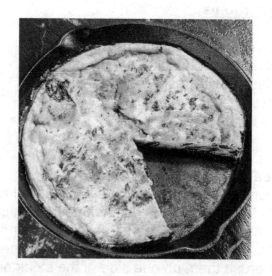

Preparing Time: 15 minutes,
Cooking Time: 35 minutes
Serving: 3 people's

Ingredients

- 5 slices of mushrooms
- 1 cup of mushrooms thinly sliced
- 3 tablespoons of melted butter
- 1 cup of finely chopped baby spinach
- 6 golden eggs
- 3 tablespoons of heavy whipping cream
- Some pinch of salt
- Some black pepper to taste
- 1 bowl of cheddar cheese

Directions

- Preheat the oven at 180 degrees
- Take a nonstick pan, add the diced bacon, then dice them for about 5 minutes. Then add the mushrooms for about 3 minutes while continuously stirring them
- Add the baby spinach in the same pan and saute them for 5 minutes
- Sprinkle the cheddar cheese in the pan and saute them with the rest of the ingredients until well combined
- Take a bowl, add golden eggs, heavy whipping cream, some salt and black pepper to taste. Whisk them together until well combined
- Now pour this whisked egg mixture in the pan and then place them in the oven.
- Bake them for about 20 minutes
- Them after 20 minutes remove them and slice them into 4 pieces
- Enjoy

Keto Herbs Omelette

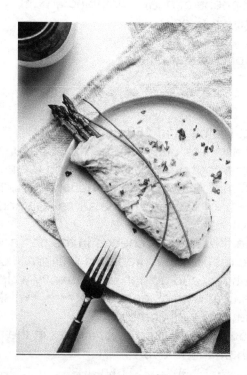

Preparing Time: 5 minutes,

Cooking Time: 5 minutes
Serving: 2 people's

Ingredients

- 2 golden eggs
- 1 tablespoon of chopped parsley
- Some kosher salt to taste
- 1 tablespoon of chives
- 3 medium-sized asparagus spear
- 2 tablespoons of avocado oil

Directions

- Take a bowl, crack eggs and herbs whisk them together until well combined
- Take a nonstick pan, drizzle some avocado oil, pour some egg
- Cook them until it is cooked
- Then sprinkle some more herbs and asparagus spear and let it cook for 2 minutes and then microwave for about 5 minutes in the oven
- Then serve it and enjoy

Keto Lettuce Cups

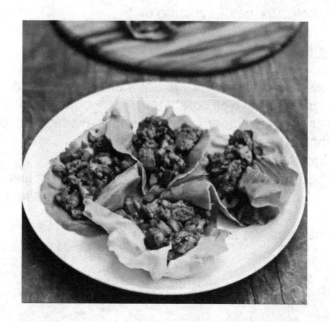

Preparing Time: 15 minutes,
Cooking Time: 10 minutes
Serving: 6 people

Ingredients

- 1 pound of ground chicken
- 1 cup of finely chopped onion
- Some kosher salt to taste
- Some ground black pepper to taste
- 3 tablespoons of canned water chestnuts chopped
- 2 green onions thinly chopped
- 1 head of bibb lettuce cups

Ingredients For Homemade Hoisin Sauce

- 5 tablespoons of soy sauce
- 2 tablespoons of natural peanut butter
- 2 tablespoons of minced garlic cloves
- 2 tablespoons of sriracha sauce
- 2 tablespoons of sesame oil
- 2 tablespoons of rice wine vinegar
- 1 teaspoon of garlic powder
- 1 teaspoon of zero calories sweetener
- Some sea salt to taste
- Some black pepper to taste

Directions

- Combine all the ingredients of homemade hoisin sauce and stir them to combine well
- Heat up the skillet and put the boneless ground chicken and sprinkle some salt and black pepper. Stir them to combine well
- Cook the chicken for about 5 minutes until well combined
- Then add the onions and hoisin sauce Cook them for about 5 minutes until the onions are tendered and

golden brown
- Now put the filling into the lettuce cups. Top them with the green onions.
- Serve them and enjoy

Keto Spaghetti

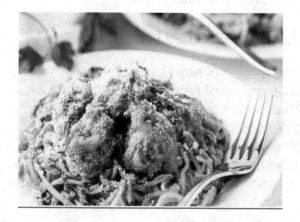

Preparing Time: 20 minutes,
Cooking Time: 30 minutes
Serving: 6 people

Ingredients

- 40 ounces of zucchini noodles

Meatball Ingredients

4 tablespoons of grated Parmesan cheese
- 2 tablespoons of Italian seasoning
- Some kosher salt to taste
- Some ground black pepper to taste
- 3 tablespoons of heavy cream
- 2 tablespoons of chopped onions
- 1 large egg
- 2 cloves of minced garlic
- 1 tablespoon of freshly chopped parsley
- 4 lbs of ground beef

Assembly

- 1 cup 9f marina sauce
- 2 tablespoons of grated Parmesan cheese

Directions

- Preheat the air fryer basket lined with the parchment paper
- Take a bowl add all the ingredients of the meatballs and mix them by using your hands. Take a cookie scoop and take the meat into your hands and make meatballs by using your hands
- Place them on the parchment lined air fryer basket and cook them for 10 minutes
- And till then cook the zucchini noodles by placing deep skillet and adding water

- Cooking them for about 7 minutes
- Then after 7 minutes drain the zucchini noodles from the skillet and place then in the bowl after draining excess water
- Remove the meatballs from the air fryer basket and set them aside. Dry the excess oil of the meat balls by using paper towel
- Now take an oven safe bowl and add the marina sauce ingredients
- Let them microwave for 1 minute
- Take a plate, add the zucchini noodles, drizzle some marina sauce and top with meatballs. Sprinkle some grated Parmesan cheese herbs
- Enjoy

Keto Chicken Salad

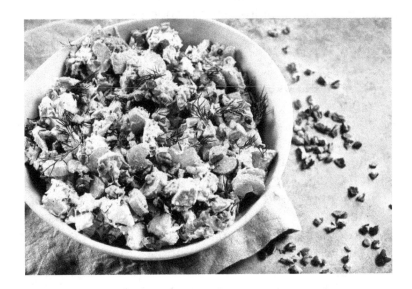

Preparing Time: 15 minutes,
Cooking Time: 30 minutes
Serving: 6 people

Ingredients

- 1 lbs of chicken thighs
- 3 ribs of celery diced
- 3 tablespoons of mayonnaise
- 2 tablespoons of brown mustard
- Some Himalayan salt to taste
- 2 tablespoons of freshly chopped dill
- 3 tablespoons of freshly chopped pecans

Directions

- Preheat the oven to 180 F, lined with the parchment paper
- Place the chicken breast on the parchment paper and bake them for about, 15 minutes
- After 15 minutes remove the chicken from the oven and let it cool. After that cut the chicken into pieces
- Take a bowl and add chicken pieces, mayonnaise, diced celery, brown mustard and some salt. Toss the ingredients together until well combined. Then cover the bowl with a plastic wrap and let them refrigerate for 2 hours
- After 2 hours remove the plastic cover and sprinkle the chopped pecans and dill
- Lightly toss then and serve chilled
- Enjoy

Keto Cheese Burger

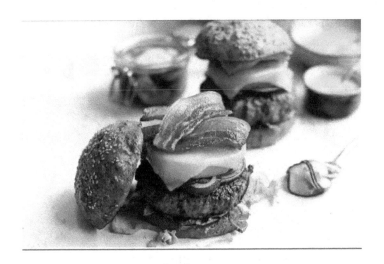

Preparing Time: 25 minutes,
Cooking Time: 25 minutes
Serving: 1 people

Ingredients

- 600 grams of ground beef
- 1 clove of minced garlic
- 2 tablespoons of onion powder
- 1 tablespoon of apple cider vinegar
- Some kosher salt to taste
- Some black pepper to taste
- 1 teaspoon of melted butter for greasing

Burger Sauce

- 4 tablespoons of mayonnaise
- 2 tablespoon of sugar-free
- 1 tablespoon of lemon juice
- Some kosher salt to taste
- Some ground black pepper to taste

Burgers

- 4 keto buns
- 2 teaspoons of melted butter
- 4 slices of bacon cut into half sized
- 2 cups of green shredded lettuce
- 9 slices of onions
- 18 slices of sugar-free pickles
- 4 slices of cheddar cheese

Directions

- Preheat the nonstick pan and prepare the keto buns. Brush the buns with egg yolks and some water to give them a shinny finish

- Take a bowl and add the Burger King patties ingredients mix then by using your hands. Don't overmix them and let them smooth
- Wet your hands and make 4 equal sizes thick burger patties
- Then by using fork pierce the patties and so that they don't get tough
- Now take a bowl add the burger sauce and stir them continuously until they are well combined
- Now place the keto buns in the pan and cook them until they are tendered or crispy
- Remove them from the skillet and then set aside
- Then in the same pan drizzle some melted butter and cook the patties for about 10 minutes until they are tendered or crispy brown
- Remove them and serve aside
- Then in the same pan add the bacon slices, cook them until they are tendered or crispy brown
- Now assemble the burger spread the sauce put the pickles and spread some shredded lettuce
- Now put the burger pattie, sliced tomatoes and cheese slice. Place this burger in the broiler and let it inside them for 1 minute
- Place the bacon slices and top them with burger bun serve them and enjoy

Low Carbs Cauliflower Pizza

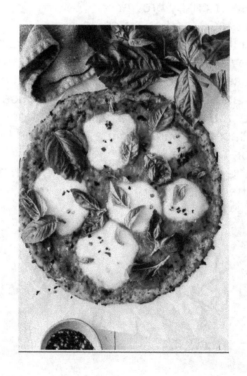

Preparing Time: 15 minutes,
Cooking Time: 25 minutes
Serving: 4 people

Ingredients

- 2 pounds of cauliflower florets
- 4 tablespoons of cream cheese
- 4 tablespoons of shredded cheese
- 1 golden egg beaten
- 1 tablespoon of Italian seasoning
- Some salt to taste
- Some ground black pepper to taste

Pesto Pizza

- 5 tablespoons of pesto sauce
- ½ cup of shredded chicken
- 3 cups of shredded mozzarella cheese
- 2 cups of baby spinach
- 2 cloves of minced garlic

Margherita Pizza

- 5 tablespoons of marina sauce
- 4 ounces of mozzarella balls, sliced
- Some fresh basil leaves
- Some red pepper flakes

Directions

- Preheat the oven at 400 degrees
- Take a food processor and add the cauliflower florets and process them
- Now add these processed cauliflower rice in an ovenproof bowl and microwave them for 3 minutes until they are softened

- Now take a thin kitchen towel and add the cauliflower rice in then squeeze the excess moisture present in the cauliflower rice
- Now after squeezing the water put the cauliflower rice in the bowl and add cheese, eggs and the rest of the seasonings. Make pizza dough by using your hands
- Now take a baking sheet lined with parchment paper and press the dough on them evenly like a pizza dough about 9 inches
- Microwave them for 25 minutes until it turns golden brown and crispy
- Now add the toppings and bake them for 10 minutes
- Then serve them and enjoy

Keto Smoofhies

Keto Strawberry Smoothie

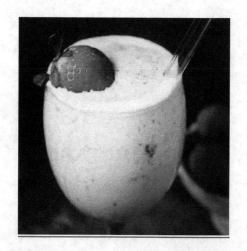

Preparing Time: 5 minutes,
Cooking Time: 3 minutes
Serving: 2 people's

Ingredients

- ½ cup of heavy whipping cream
- 3 cups of unsweetened almond milk
- 1 tablespoon of granulated stevia
- 2 cups of frozen strawberries
- ½ cup of ice
- ½ teaspoon of vanilla extract

Directions

- Take a blender and add all the ingredients together until well combined and smoothie creamy smoothie formed
- Serve chilled

Keto Peanut Butter Smoothie

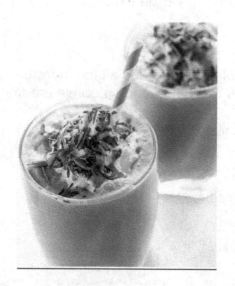

Preparing Time: 5 minutes,
Cooking Time: 3 minutes S
erving: 2 people's

Ingredients

- 4 tablespoon of peanut butter
- 1 tablespoon of cocoa powder
- ¼ cup of heavy whipping cream
- 3 cups of unsweetened almond milk
- 5 tablespoon of besti powdered erythritol
- Some pinch of salt to taste

Directions

- Take a blender and blend all the ingredients together until well combined and smooth creamy smoothie is formed
- Serve chilled

Green Keto Smoothie

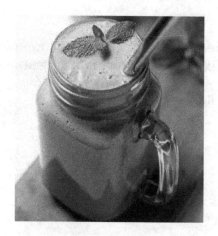

Preparing Time: 5 minutes,
Cooking Time: 3 minutes
Serving: 2 people's

Ingredients

- 1 cup of kale leaves
- ½ avocado peeled and seed removed
- 1 stick of celery chopped
- ½ cucumber peeled and chopped
- 1 cup of unsweetened almond milk
- 1 tablespoon of almond butter
- 2 tablespoons of lemon juice

Directions

- Take a blender and blend all the ingredients together until well combined and creamy smoothie forms

Keto Blueberry Smoothie

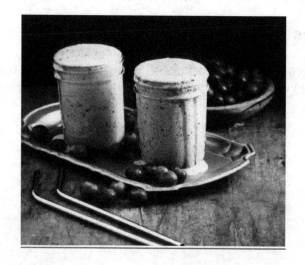

Preparing Time: 5 minutes,
Cooking Time: 3 minutes
Serving: 2 people's

Ingredients

- ¼ cup of heavy whipping cream
- 3 cups of unsweetened almond milk
- ½ cup of cream cheese
- 2 tablespoons of granulated stevia
- ½ cup of blueberries
- 1 scoop of peptides
- ½ cup of ice
- ½ teaspoon of vanilla extract
- 5 drops of lemon juice

Directions

- Take a blender and blend all the ingredients together until well combined and creamy smoothie forms
- Serve chilled

Coconut Chocolate Keto Smoothie

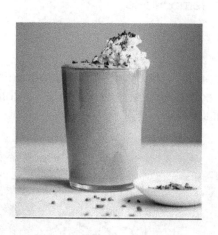

Preparing Time: 5 minutes,
Cooking Time: 3 minutes
Serving: 2 people's

Ingredients

- ½ avocado slices and seed removed
- 2 cups of almond milk
- ¼ cup of heavy whipping cream
- 1 teaspoon of chia seeds
- 1 tablespoon of cocoa powder
- 1 teaspoon of extra virgin olive oil
- 1 tablespoon of almond butter
- 1 teaspoon of extra collagen protein
- 1 teaspoon of sweetener
- 1 tablespoon of heavy whipping cream
- 1 tablespoon of cocoa powder for topping

Directions

- Take a blender and add all the ingredients in a blender and blend them until creamy smoothie forms
- Serve chilled

Keto Mint And Strawberry Smoothie

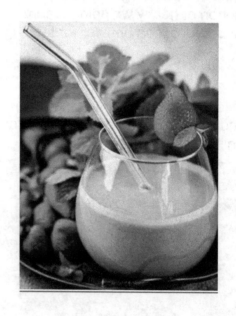

Preparing Time: 5 minutes,
Cooking Time: 3 minutes
Serving: 2 people's

Ingredients

- ½ cup of mint leaves
- 1 cup of frozen strawberries
- 1 cup of almond milk
- 2 tablespoons of heavy cream
- ⅛ teaspoon of chia seeds
- ½ teaspoon of collagen powder
- 5 drops of lemon juice
- 1 tablespoon of peanut butter
- ½ cup of ice

Directions

- Take a blender and add all the ingredients together until well combined and blend them until creamy smoothie forms
- Serve chilled

Cucumber Spinach Smoothie

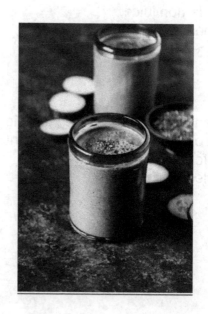

Preparing Time: 5 minutes,
Cooking Time: 3 minutes

Serving: 2 people's

Ingredients

- 1 whole cucumber peeled and diced
- 2 cups of baby spinach
- 1 cup of almond milk
- 1 cup of iced water
- 1 teaspoon of chia seeds
- 1 tablespoon of agave nectar
- 5 ice cubes
- ½ teaspoon of Stevia sweetener

Directions

- Take a blender and blend all the ingredients together in a blender until smooth creamy smoothie forms
- Serve chilled

Keto Avocado Green Smoothie

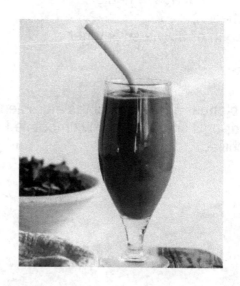

Preparing Time: 5 minutes,
Cooking Time: 3 minutes
Serving: 2 people's

Ingredients

- 1 cup of Kale
- 1 cup of almond milk
- 1 teaspoon of Lemon juice
- 1 avocado peeled, seed removed and diced
- 1 tablespoon of protein powder
- 1 tablespoon of peanut butter
- ½ teaspoon of cinnamon powder
- 6-7 baby spinach leaves

Directions

- Take a blender and blend all the ingredients together until well combined and smooth creamy smoothie forms
- Serve chilled

Pineapple And Kale Smoothie

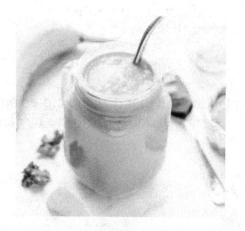

Preparing Time: 5 minutes,
Cooking Time: 3 minutes
Serving: 2 people's

Ingredients

- 2 cups of finely chopped
- 3 cups of unsweetened vanilla milk
- 2 frozen bananas (cut into chunks)
- ¼ cup of Greek yogurt
- ½ cup of frozen pineapples cut into cubes
- 2 tablespoons of peanut butter
- 1 tablespoon of honey

Directions

- Take a blended and add all the ingredients together until well combined and smooth creamy smoothie is formed
- Serve chilled

Mango And Avocado Keto Smoothie

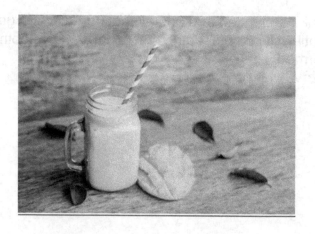

Preparing Time: 5 minutes,
Cooking Time: 3 minutes
Serving: 2 people's

Ingredients

- 1 cup of frozen banana peeled and diced
- ½ avocado sliced and seed removed
- 1 teaspoon of unsweetened cup of almond milk
- 1 teaspoon of Lemon juice
- ¼ cup of water
- 1 teaspoon of sugar

Directions

- Take a blended and add all the ingredients together until well combined and smooth creamy smoothie is formed
- Serve chilled

Conclusion

Thank you, my readers, for making it to the end!

9 781802 940442